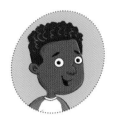

In Our Neighborhood

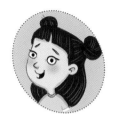

Meet a Doctor!

by AnnMarie Anderson

Illustrations by Lisa Hunt

Children's Press®
An imprint of Scholastic Inc.

SCHOLASTIC

Special thanks to our content consultants:

Nishant Magar, MD
Jamie Abatemarco, RN
Kelly A. Mayo, RN, BSN, CEN

Library of Congress Cataloging-in-Publication Data
Names: Anderson, AnnMarie, author. | Hunt, Lisa, 1973– illustrator.
Title: In our neighborhood. Meet a doctor! / by AnnMarie Anderson; [illustrations by Lisa Hunt].
Other titles: Meet a doctor!
Description: New York: Children's Press, an imprint of Scholastic Inc., 2021. | Series: In our neighborhood |
    Includes index. | Audience: Ages 5–7. | Audience: Grades K–1. | Summary: "Two children learn the
    importance of doctors in their community"— Provided by publisher.
Identifiers: LCCN 2020031733 | ISBN 9780531136836 (library binding) | ISBN 9780531136898 (paperback)
Subjects: LCSH: Physicians—Juvenile literature. | Hospitals—Emergency services—Juvenile literature.
Classification: LCC R690 .H48 2021 | DDC 610.69/5—dc23
LC record available at https://lccn.loc.gov/2020031733

Produced by Spooky Cheetah Press
Prototype design by Maria Bergós/Book & Look
Page design by Kathleen Petelinsek/The Design Lab

Printed in North Mankato, MN, USA 113

1 2 3 4 5 6 7 8 9 10 R 30 29 28 27 26 25 24 23 22 21

Scholastic Inc., 557 Broadway, New York, NY 10012.

Photos ©: 7 top: Todd Bannor/Alamy Images; 9: Sasiistock/Getty Images;
11: Chris Bjornberg/Science Source; 12 left: Steve Hix/Fuse/Getty Images; 12 right:
KidStock/Getty Images; 13 left: SDI Productions/Getty Images; 15: xavierarnau/
Getty Images; 16: SDI Productions/Getty Images; 18: shapecharge/Getty Images;
22: xavierarnau/Getty Images; 25: SDI Productions/Getty Images; 31 bottom left:
Vladyslav Danilin/Getty Images.

All other photos © Shutterstock.

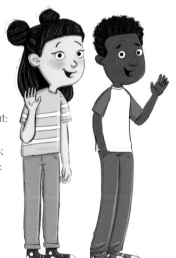

Table of Contents

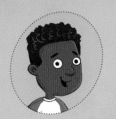
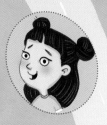

OUR NEIGHBORHOOD

Hi! I'm Theo. This is my best friend, Emma. Welcome to our neighborhood!

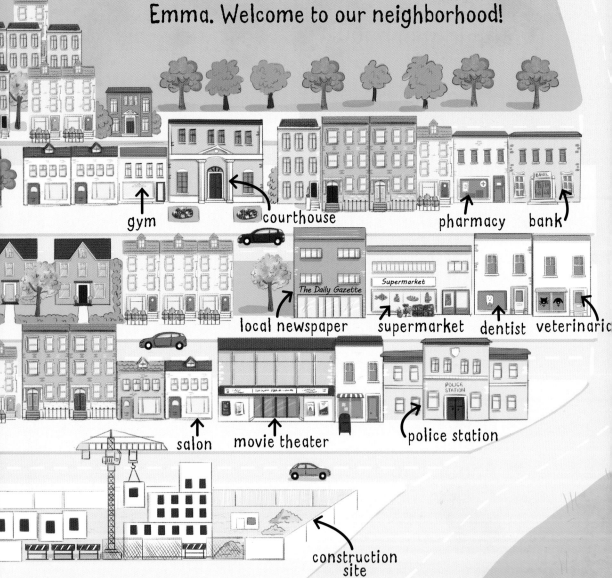

gym

courthouse

pharmacy

bank

local newspaper

supermarket

dentist

veterinaria

salon

movie theater

police station

construction site

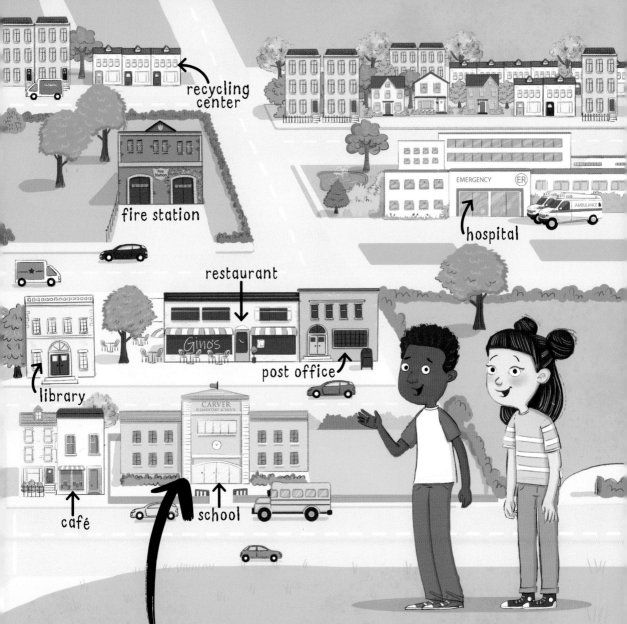

recycling center

fire station

hospital

restaurant

post office

library

café

school

Our school is right there. Emma and I love to play soccer there. The other day we were warming up, and I got hurt pretty badly.

GOING TO THE HOSPITAL

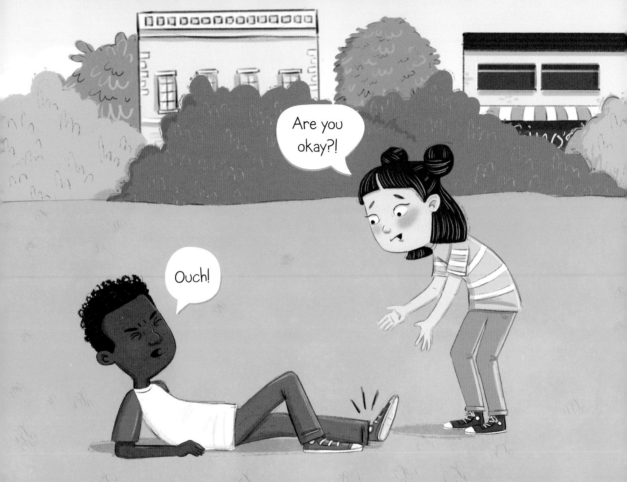

I dribbled the ball down the field. Then, as I kicked the ball toward the goal, I slipped and fell.

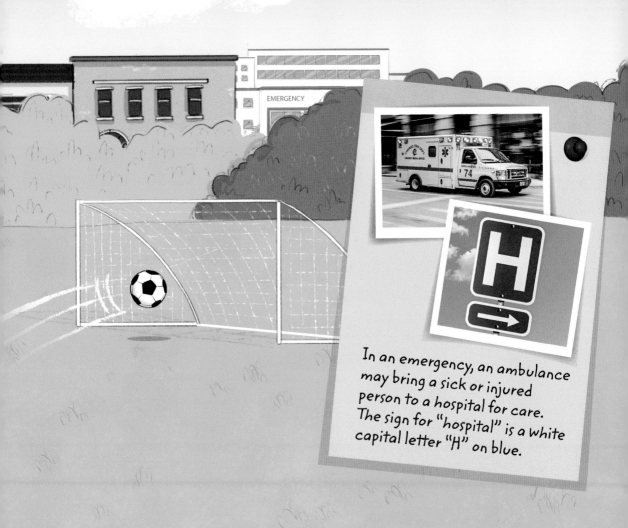

In an emergency, an ambulance may bring a sick or injured person to a hospital for care. The sign for "hospital" is a white capital letter "H" on blue.

My ankle hurt. A lot. Luckily, Emma's mom was there. She said I needed a doctor. She called my dad and asked him to meet us at the hospital emergency room.

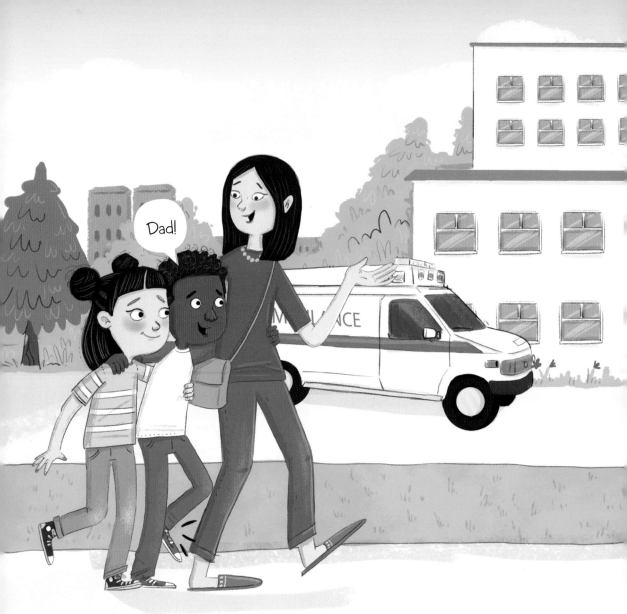

I was so glad to see my dad! I was nervous.
I had never been to a hospital. When I go to the
doctor, it's usually for a checkup with Dr. Clark.

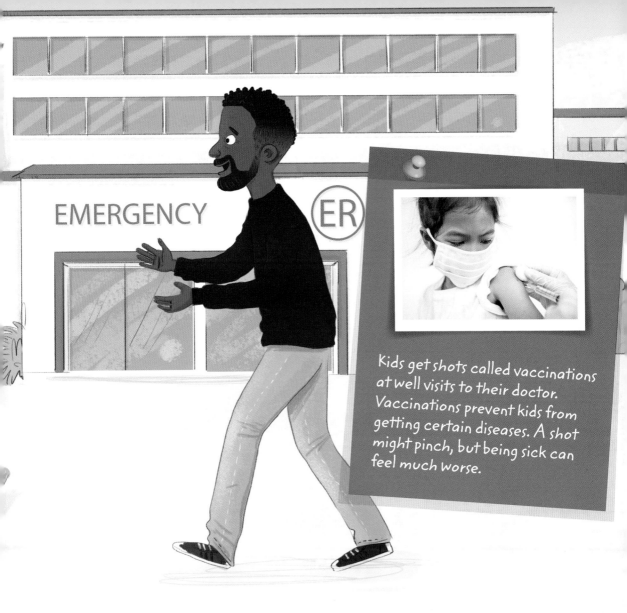

Kids get shots called vaccinations at well visits to their doctor. Vaccinations prevent kids from getting certain diseases. A shot might pinch, but being sick can feel much worse.

Dr. Clark measures my height and weight to see how I am growing. He looks in my eyes and ears. He listens to my heart and lungs. Sometimes I get a shot, but it's not so bad.

I didn't know what to expect in the emergency room. First a nurse took my information. Then I told her what happened to my foot.

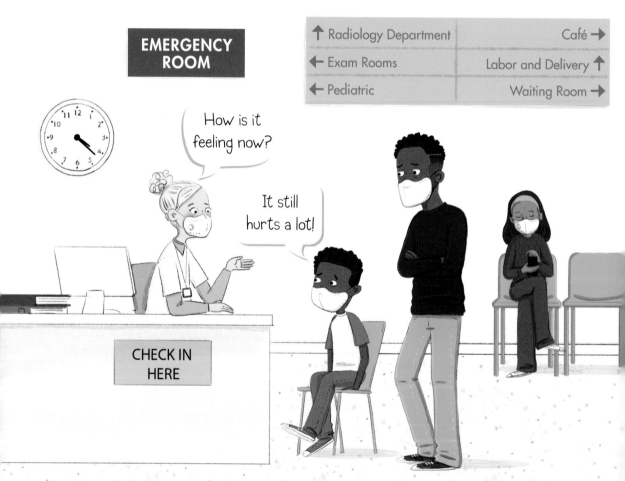

Another nurse used a thermometer to check my temperature. She checked my vital signs. Then she gave me ice to put on my ankle.

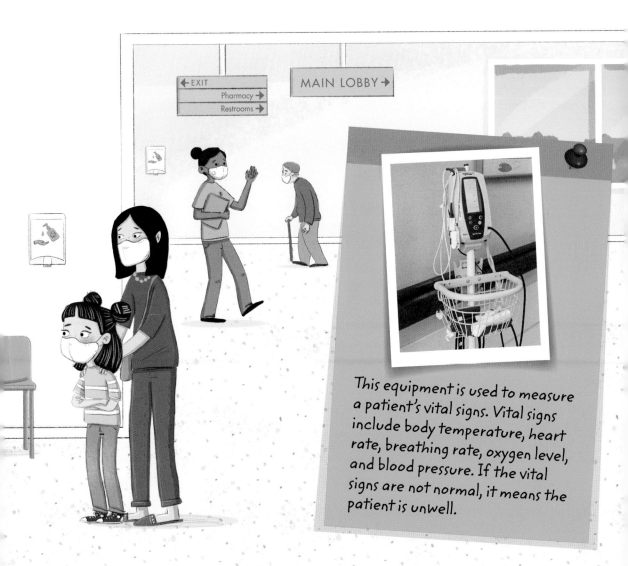

This equipment is used to measure a patient's vital signs. Vital signs include body temperature, heart rate, breathing rate, oxygen level, and blood pressure. If the vital signs are not normal, it means the patient is unwell.

"Many doctors work at a hospital," my dad explained while we waited. "Some work in the emergency room. Some deliver babies. And some work in the operating room. They are called surgeons."

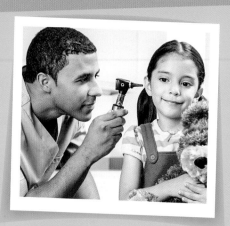

A **pediatrician** is a doctor who cares for kids.

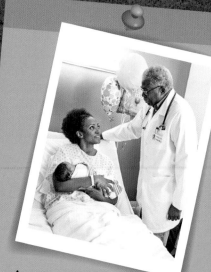

An **obstetrician** cares for pregnant women and their newborn babies.

Did the surgery hurt

"I had an operation once!" Emma told us. "The surgeon put tubes in my ears so I would hear better."

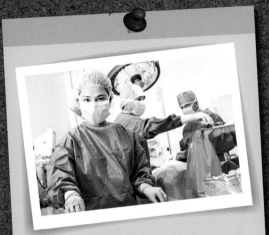

A **surgeon** performs operations.

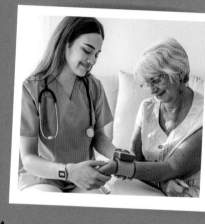

A **cardiologist** takes care of the heart and blood vessels.

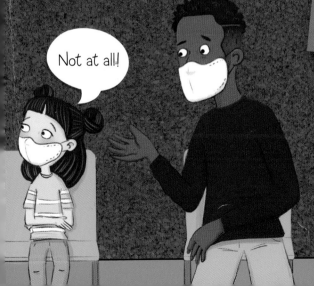

Not at all!

MEET DR. GÓMEZ

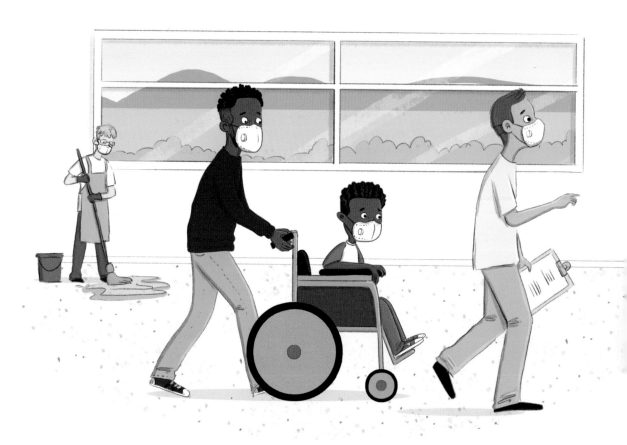

Soon a different nurse called my name. My dad and I followed him to an exam room. I changed into a gown.

A few minutes later, Dr. Gómez arrived. She asked me how I got hurt.

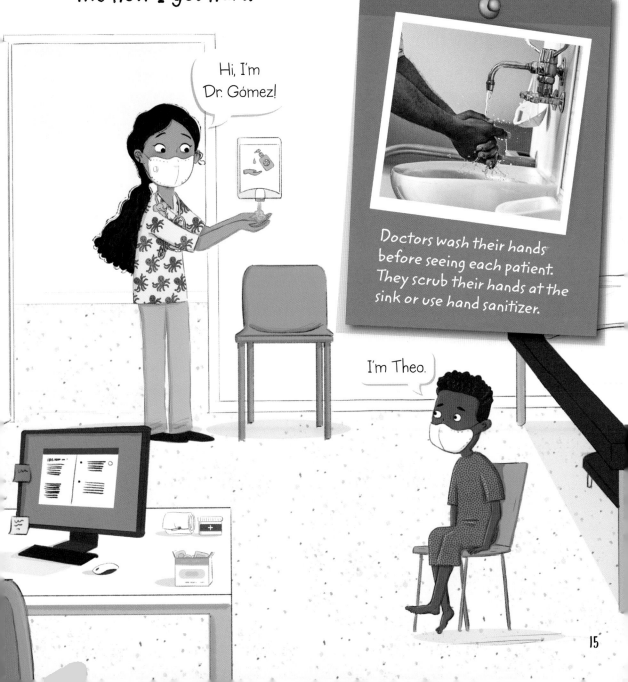

Hi, I'm Dr. Gómez!

Doctors wash their hands before seeing each patient. They scrub their hands at the sink or use hand sanitizer.

I'm Theo.

Dr. Gómez said she was going to examine me. She wanted to be sure my ankle was my only injury. Dr. Gómez listened to my heart and lungs with her stethoscope. She looked in my eyes. She checked my neck and spine.

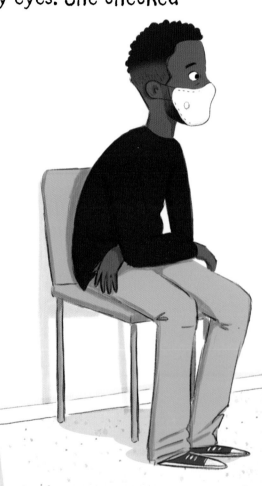

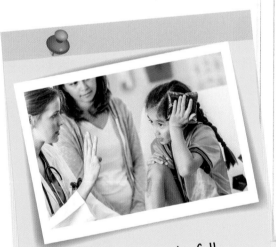

If a patient has had a fall, the doctor will check for a concussion. That's a serious head injury.

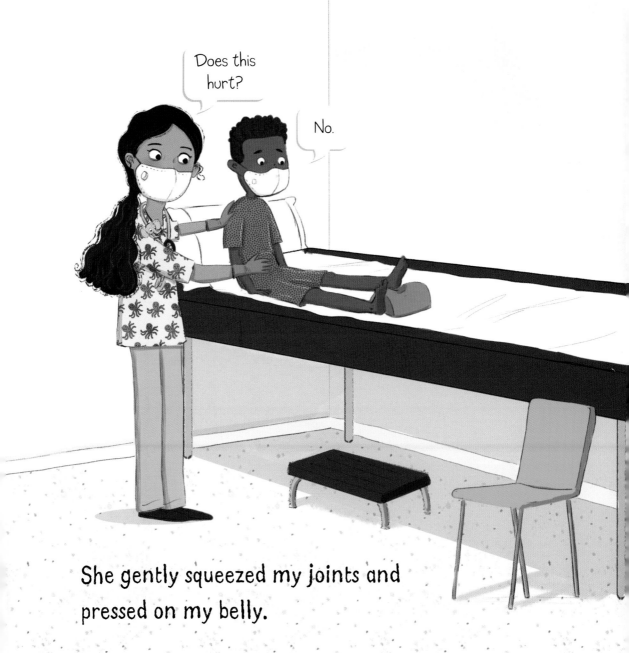

She gently squeezed my joints and
pressed on my belly.

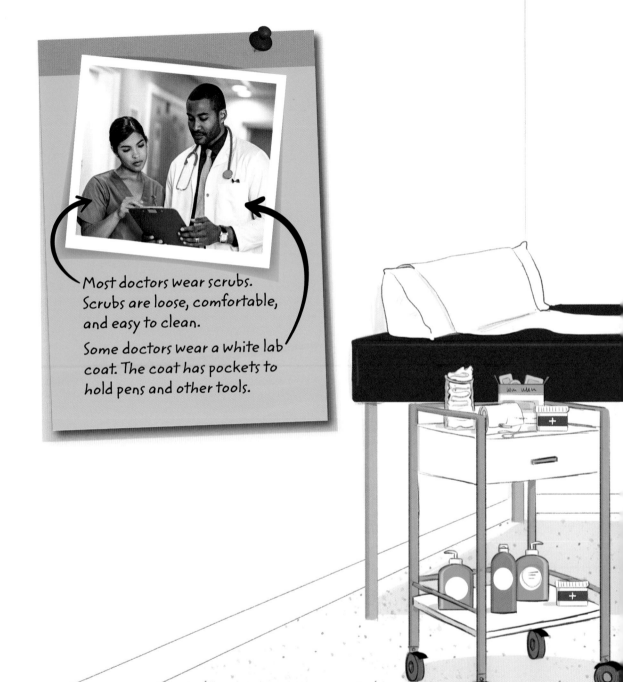

Most doctors wear scrubs. Scrubs are loose, comfortable, and easy to clean.

Some doctors wear a white lab coat. The coat has pockets to hold pens and other tools.

Dr. Gómez noticed a cut on my knee. She cleaned it and put on a bandage.

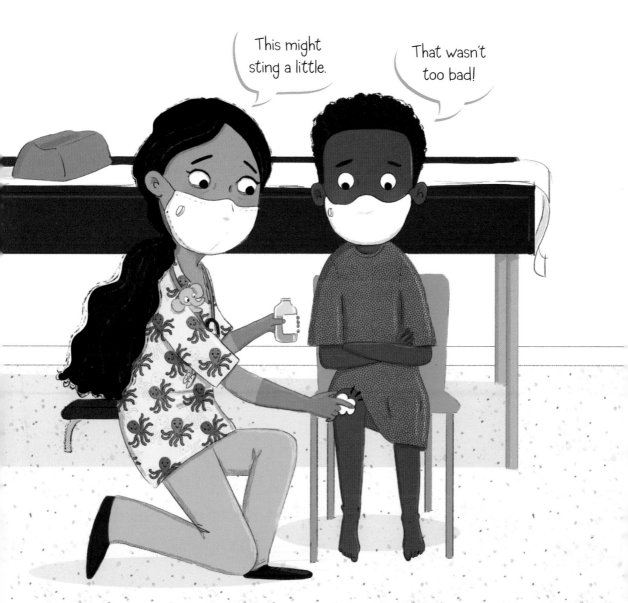

Next Dr. Gómez touched
my foot gently.

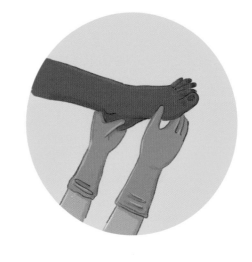

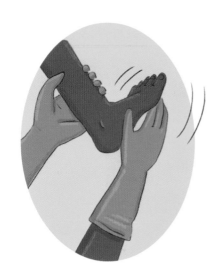

She moved my ankle
from left to right.

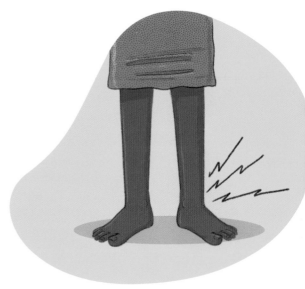

Then she asked if I could
stand on my foot. I couldn't.
It hurt too much.

Dr. Gómez told me I needed to get an X-ray. That would show if a bone was broken.

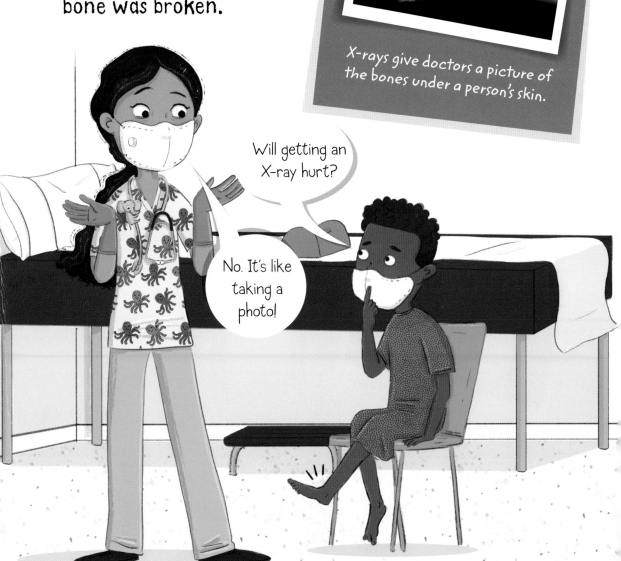

X-rays give doctors a picture of the bones under a person's skin.

Will getting an X-ray hurt?

No. It's like taking a photo!

GETTING AN X-RAY

My dad and I went to the radiology department.
A technician named Oscar asked me to lie down.

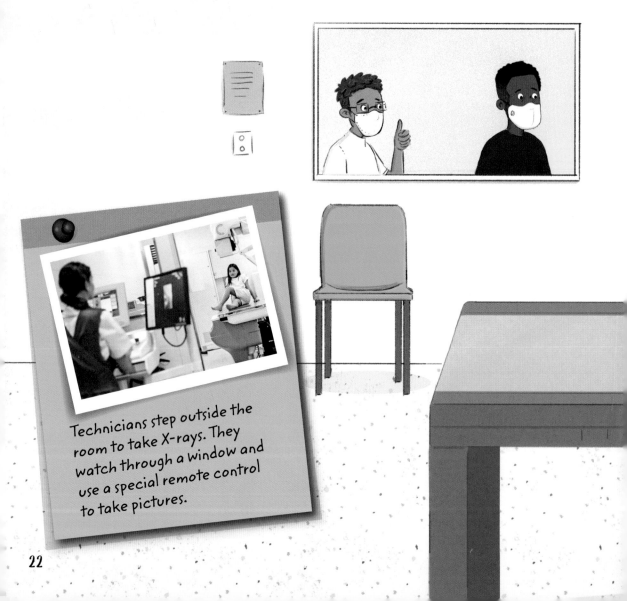

Technicians step outside the room to take X-rays. They watch through a window and use a special remote control to take pictures.

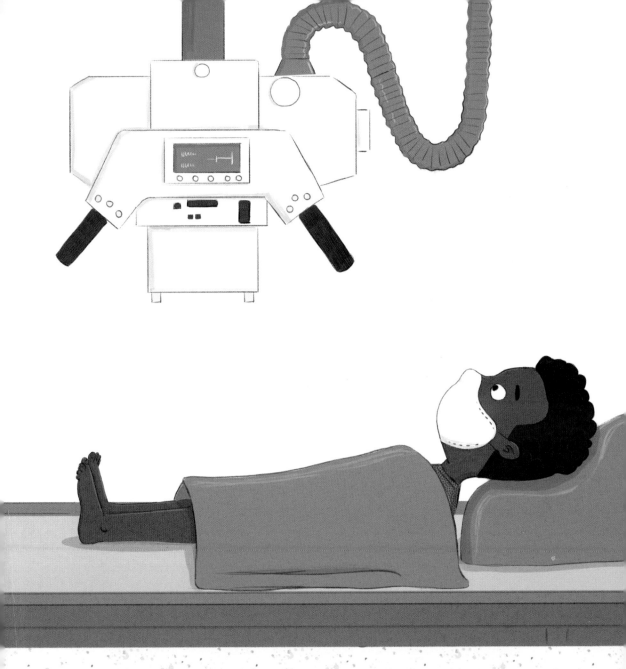

Oscar put a heavy lead apron over the top of my body. Then he asked me to keep my foot still.

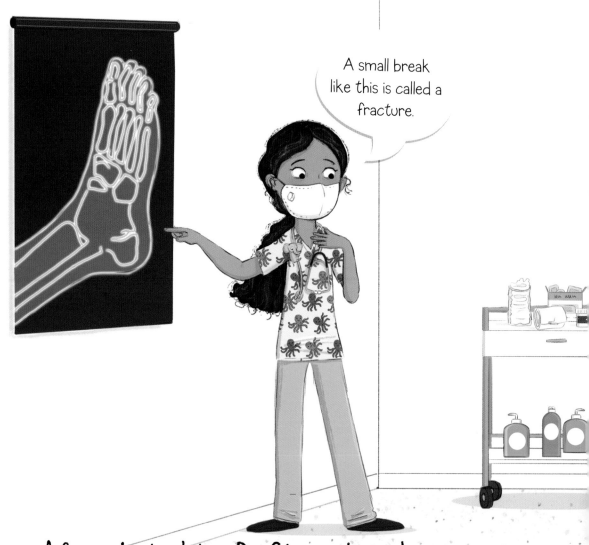

A small break like this is called a fracture.

A few minutes later, Dr. Gómez showed me my X-ray. She said I had a small break in a bone in my ankle.

Dr. Gómez told me I would have to see another doctor in two weeks. The orthopedist would make sure my foot was healing. I would also have to wear a special boot for six weeks.

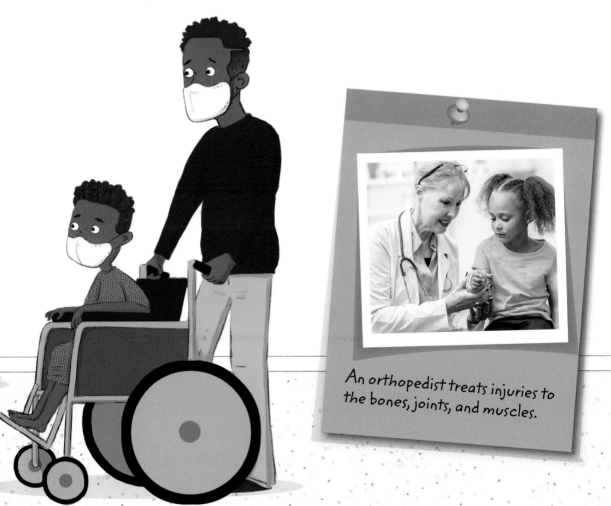

An orthopedist treats injuries to the bones, joints, and muscles.

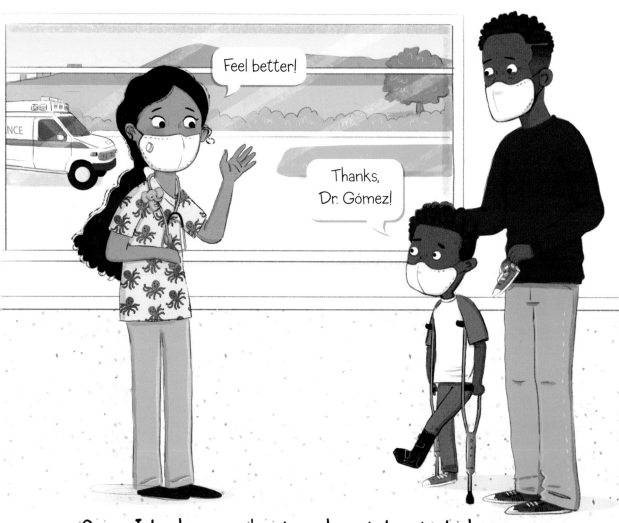

Soon I had a new boot and crutches to help me
get around. When I left the exam room, Emma
was waiting for me.

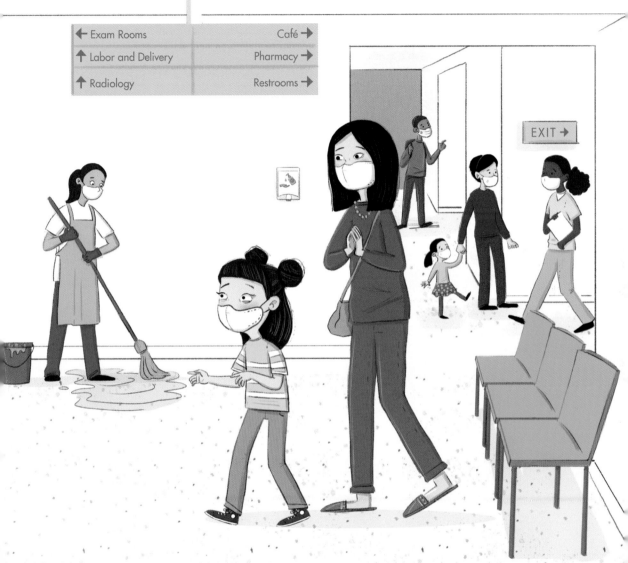

Exam Rooms ←
Café →
↑ Labor and Delivery
Pharmacy →
↑ Radiology
Restrooms →

EXIT →

"Don't worry," I told her. "It looks bad, but I'll be okay. Dr. Gómez said I'll be playing soccer again in no time!"

Ask a Doctor

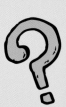
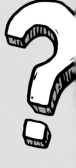

Emma asked Dr. Gómez about her job as a pediatric doctor in the emergency room.

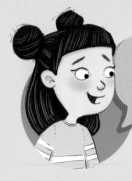

How many years did you study to become a doctor?

Twelve years. I spent four years in college and four years in medical school. Then I spent four years as a resident in an emergency room. Being a resident was like on-the-job training!

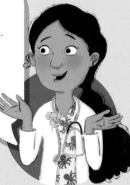

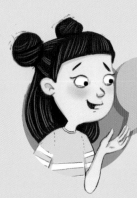

Do you work at night?

Yes. I work in 12-hour shifts, and sometimes those are at night.

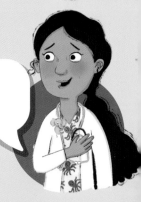

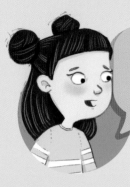

What are some reasons kids come to the emergency room other than broken bones?

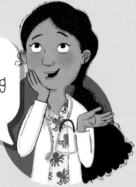

Fevers, rashes, and very deep cuts are common. A deep cut is one that is bleeding too much for a regular bandage.

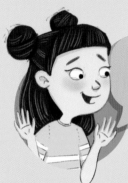

How many kids do you see each day?

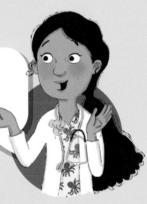

It depends. Some days I'll see 10 patients, and other days I'll see as many as 30.

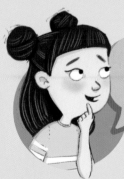

What is your favorite thing about your job?

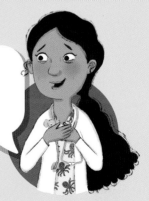

I'm trained to know what to do in an emergency, and I love knowing I've helped a child feel better.

Dr. Gómez's Tips for Staying Healthy

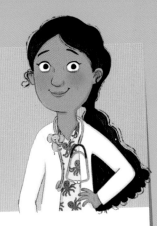

- Wash your hands often, for at least 20 seconds each time.

- Always cough or sneeze into your elbow—not your hands.

- Keep your body active with regular exercise.

- Drink lots of water and eat nutritious foods.

- Wear a mask when necessary or required.

- Get plenty of sleep every night.

- Visit your doctor for a checkup once a year.

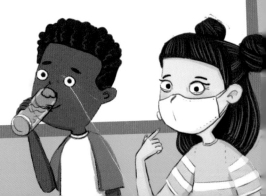

A Doctor's Tools

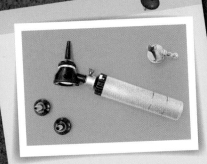

Otoscope: Doctors use this tool to look inside the ears and nose.

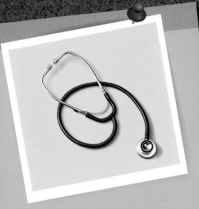

Stethoscope: Doctors use this instrument to listen to the heart and lungs.

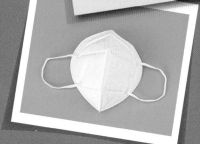

Mask: Doctors wear this covering over the nose and mouth.

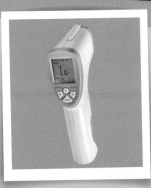

Thermometer: Doctors use this tool to measure a patient's temperature.

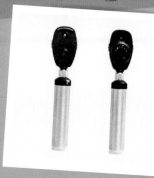

Ophthalmoscope: Doctors use this tool to look into the eyes.

Index

About the Author

AnnMarie Anderson has written numerous books for young readers—from easy readers to novels. She lives in Brooklyn, New York, with her husband and sons, where she tries her best to stay out of the emergency room!